LATE ON THE ROAD OF LIFE

I MET A MAN NAMED

PARKINSON:

A Conversation

Eugene P. Clemens

ISBN 978-0-9977956-2-2

Published in the United States by Yesteryear Publishing.

Books are available at www.amazon.com as well as through the author or publisher:

Yesteryear Publishing
P.O. Box 311
Hummelstown, PA 17036

www.yesteryearpublishing.com
yesteryearpublishing@gmail.com
(717) 566-3907

Author:

Eugene P. Clemens. Native of Indiana. M. A. in Philosophy, Ph.D. in Religious Thought, University of Pennsylvania. Professor Emeritus, Religious Studies, Elizabethtown College, 1965-2000. Mentor and Photographer, Men's Soccer Team. Diagnosed with Parkinson's, 2010.

Editor:

Judith T. Witmer, Ed.D., Principal, Yesteryear Publishing

Designer:

E. Nan Edmunds, Yesteryear Publishing

DEDICATION

This journal of honest confession is dedicated to all those who have been chosen by blind fate to walk the road with Parkinson's Disease. Thus, it is an "inside job," a sincere communiqué to those similarly afflicted.

Truly there is company on a common path, different as the life particulars and personality peculiarities may be. Fellow travelers, I do understand.

The purpose of compiling these daily reflections is twofold:

1. that my family may better understand what I was undergoing within, as they watched the external effect of Parkinson's; and

2. that others who may be afflicted with Parkinson's Disease may become acquainted with what to expect in their own experience.

The universal truth of human existence is that we share it and that experience is more than what is seen on the surface.

To all I extend the compassion only empathy can bestow.

PREFACE

My life journey has been long and eventful. Curiosity led me by the hand as a child, to be taken over by the compelling need to be in union with life. The travel through space and time, compassion and friendship, passion and love, has left me with enormous and varied experiences, only later peppered with difficulties. One thing I have learned is that the road goes ever on.

In the midst of a life full of positive and loving experiences, a specter of infirmity took its place beside me; in slow but increasing awareness, he tapped me on my right side, insisting that he accompany me from then on. I preferred that he did not.

However, the power of his insistence was undeniable and I accepted that his companionship was unavoidable. No longer was the question, "How do I evade him?" Rather, I was left with the question, "How do I relate to him?"

He gave me his name. It was Parkinson.

At times I have resented his persistent presence, for how he has stolen from me the vigor and enthusiasm of youth. Remaining is the impulse to give him an imaginary brush-off, in the most cold shoulder manner possible. But his attendance is constant; I cannot elude him.

I refuse to confuse his name with mine. My dignity forbids that loss of identity. My sense of fairness refuses to complain of life's undesired fortuity. With so much given me in more than my share of years, what right do I possess to demand special favor?

Yes, I have enjoyed many years, many miles, and the support of many loved ones. The vessel of my selfhood has been filled to overflowing with goodness. Who am I to deny that, even in the face of old age? Though I hold Parkinson largely responsible for the diminishing of my strength, I know that he serves a double character. His gaunt figure is also the profile of senility. Age is prefigured in Parkinson. The two are working simultaneously to render me strengthless and senile; in a word, the object is to make me the Old One.

Unable to deny Parkinson's inseparable company, I eventually worked out an agreement. Negotiations came to this: I chose to allow his presence only for what it could teach me about life. It seemed my graduate degree in wisdom had yet another course for completion. Full wisdom has many chapters and numerous degrees. Thus, I shall not fail my appointed rendezvous with understanding. With this, I became more disposed to listen and learn, to hear and to love.

What follows are spontaneous thoughts occurring in the course of a year's realization of Parkinson's presence. Prior to the diagnosis one February day, I had suffered the symptoms unaware of the cause, somewhat oblivious to the degree of decline. A year before, my dear wife, Vada, had noticed that I did not swing my right arm while walking, dragging my right foot to some extent. Yet, out of kindness and perhaps not to embarrass me, she said nothing. In March of the previous year while traveling to Ireland with the college men's soccer team, it became apparent that my stamina was significantly compromised. I labored to walk any distance, with heaviness of legs and weariness of motivation.

At Christmas of that year I tripped over a chair that had been placed on its side in a doorway, to prevent a dog from entering the dining room. I was puzzled by the incident, since my mind had told my right foot to hop over the chair. Why, then, did not my foot respond accordingly? Instead, my foot caught the leg of the chair and I fell.

Slowly the reality of my condition became clear. It was time to consult my family physician who referred me to a neurologist. Subsequent to that, with medication and greater awareness, I have recognized that I am a Parkinson's patient.

I choose to keep a journal to describe the year I view as representative of the middle stage of the disease because at that point in the disease the significant degree of development allows for serious reflection. Denial is over at that point and the work of acceptance has begun. Life goes on, but with drastic modification. It is my hope that this may be a tribute to life's strong instinct.

On the Road Conversations

December 15

I stand before the door of death, one of the many calling me to reflect upon life. Not yet ready to knock, I feel death's ominous presence. Being of serious mind, I have often thought of death. Now, the question recedes from the academic, reaching down into the marrow of my bones, in ways I have not experienced before. I feel like a condemned inmate, awaiting execution. I ask myself if this could be the curse placed upon me on the road of natural aging? I repeat, I have not experienced this degree of mortality's premonition before, not in this overwhelming manner.

December 19

More earnestly than before do I reflect upon the old saying, "The spirit is willing, but the flesh is weak." The apparent point seems to be, all of our good intentions are held back by lethargy of the body. For most of my life the two have been in matched tandem, the two pulling my desires forward.

Never an overachiever, nevertheless my determination has been strong and my body has been cooperative. In my early twenties I modestly boasted of an indomitable spirit. But now, both the carriage and the driver are slowing, at times to a near stop.

To the extent I acknowledge the biological basis of the mind-body unity, I realize that aging and Parkinson's have my spirit in their grasp. I will not, however, permit them to take me captive. Until the last, I shall preserve an attitude of worth and dignity. In some kind of consolation, energy has given way to serenity.

December 24

Frankly, Parkinson, I am tired of you, for you have made me tired. You will not leave me alone. You are always there, present at my arising and residing. I did not choose you, but we have become inseparable. You go wherever I go, a constant accomplice in whatever I do. You rob me of making up my own mind. What shall I do with you?

December 28

What can I learn from you, Parkinson? You give me no answers, but you do force the question. My life experience has been enormous, yet its totality does not answer the why for my existence.

Last night I had a dream in which I was scraping heavy paper from off a wall, layer after layer. Now awake, I wonder whether this does not symbolize my search for ultimate meaning. Just as the skin protects the nerve-laden tissue of the body from daily abrasion, so does meaning shield the self from the threat of nonbeing.

So, Parkinson, I guess you will not let me free from the question. In spite of you I must answer the question of why I have existed. At your insistence clearer it has become, I have existed to absorb all that is life and to give it back as wisdom. To exhibit that truth in my living and writing is my purpose.

December 29

Aha, Parkinson, I have found you out! You are a stand-in for all the disagreeable complications in life, all that is less than what we had hoped for. Must I be angry with you, or may I go on with purpose, irrespective of you? You are not me, still I shall not regard you as an enemy. At worst, you are a reminder of my mortality and of the necessity to affirm life every day, until it comes to the time to lie down to endless sleep.

December 31

As I face a new year, what do you have in store for me, Parkinson? I will fight your "take-over" of my life. Yet, I know that my decline will continue. More activities will fall aside and each day will be more haunted by shades of decrepitude. My strength remains, "Have no fear, so long as Love is near."

January 1

So, I am to turn over a new leaf, but with a declining sense of purpose? Prospects are more limited and the pace will be slower, but more than ever on the sidelines, than in the full flow of the game. Nevertheless, I receive a new year with gratitude, if not with zest.

On the one hand, I am astonished at all that life has been—so great a reservoir of places, times, and persons—and have difficulty in knowing where to put more memory. On the other hand, I know that to accept the continuing gift of life is to renegotiate the contract of existence, and not to renegotiate would be to sever the thin line of living. I must believe that I shall further fulfill myself in the uncertainty of this coming year.

January 8

For a week I have been in the doldrums of affliction, unable to think beyond basic care for my wellbeing. A terrible cold persists in holding me captive to a mental fog, disinclined to form coherent thought. Coughing is nearly constant, aggravating a need for a quiet rest. Traces of blood in my urine, reminder of a prostate procedure from nearly three weeks ago, continues to play nervously upon Parkinson's curse of anxiety.

Whom do I blame? My fellow traveler is the likely and easy target, but I am fair enough to accept that the decline in health is the natural course of senescence, growing old. I feel so frail and vulnerable. Yet why should I complain, I have had eighty years of good living. Though my traveling companion's name could be many, I hold Parkinson as largely responsible.

January 12

Depression is another personage in Parkinson's theatre of characters. In a large percentage of cases the two come together to form one. I admit to a long history of melancholy, a penchant toward the sadder shades of reflective thought. Still, depression has taken on a different and more numbing hold with Parkinson.

It is not a death wish or suicidal temptation, but more a premonition of life's ending. Objectively the deflation of spirit can be diagnosed clinically. Subjectively, the inner encounter with depression is quite personal and pervasive. I view each day in more final terms and each night wonder about tomorrow. Plans for the future recede in priority, giving way to the immediacy of today's challenge. Depression is a thief of many faces.

January 14

I notice when Parkinson is around and talking to me, my emotions go flat, if not negative. In that regard I consider this knave a thief. Prior to his arrival I had always considered enthusiasm one of my truest friends. So tight and inseparable has been this bond that my identity is tied up with the ability to be emotional if not exuberant. How now can I sing the Hymn of Joy, if Parkinson robs me of my best attribute? It is one thing to take away my curious mind, but why my poetic heart? Will I have to make my song quieter and more subdued?

January 17

It has been a month since I took the first of three annual tests measuring Parkinson's effect upon memory. I was stunned! Yes, age has set in and senility will have its eventual toll. But, Parkinson, I hold you responsible for declining intellectual acuity. Is it not you who provides the near constant dull headache and blurred mental focus?

Not being able to connect names to clear facial features is frustrating enough. Now you are straining my ability to hold incoming information for more than a few seconds. The once clean slate, the famous tabula rasa, over a lifetime became brimming with minute details, much of which is still etched in memory.

But now, big, bold ideas are elusive. It is not a matter of will power; rather, it is a factor of sticking power. I will to focus, but get evaporation. When I am given a series of words to remember and repeat back, a fog takes over my mind until eventually mental activity actually shuts down. It is as though a "tilt button" or tripwire is set off, indicating an overload.

My mind goes on hiatus, wanting to lie down and rest. As it shuts down, the world around is shut out, leaving the impression to others of "absent mindedness." I am sure at a certain point in Parkinson's grip I will appear to be confused and out of touch with the outer world. Negotiating a day's demands will be increasingly difficult.

Ah, the vigor and ready receptivity of youth, when our minds were "steel traps," able to catch any factoid flying through the air, even when adults thought we were not listening. Again, Parkinson, you are a surrogate for aging. It is moot as to who is more responsible. The two of you seem inseparable.

January 20

Today I "burned" the season's DVD for the soccer team. Quite an accomplishment, given the heightened anxiety I experience whenever my mind is put to the task of venturing into problem solving. Even though I had accomplished the feat a year ago—with the assistance of a technician at the College, I retained little confidence that I could do it again.

Then, along with the lack of confidence loomed another resistance. With a dull headache, blurred mental focus, and diminished gumption, an unconscious reluctance sets in. If not coached with reassurance, this lack of confidence can turn into an irritability. I must teach myself not to permit annoyance to turn into anger.

After I successfully burned the project, in place of a sense of accomplishment was the relief of having it over with. Anxiety before; relief afterwards. How different the successes of youth and that of age.

January 22

The coin of looking backwards has two sides. With the complications of aging provided by my sidekick, Parkinson, I reflect upon what I have lost. I cannot run and jump anymore, as I did for hours on a basketball court. Even bicycling has slipped from my grip. Wobbly walking is an achievement nowadays. Oh, I have lost so much physically. Every year, it seems, something more is taken from me, until invalidity takes over?

But the other side of reflection's coin is the reminder that I was within my lifetime able to do what I have now lost. With a faint stir of excitement I recall body-aching football practice, somersaults off the diving board, the vigorous chopping of wood, long footloose hikes in Europe, to mention only a few. May they represent all that life used to be!

In viewing youth today I could be resentful of their freedom of activity, the vitality and energy abounding. But that would weigh down my soul more than desirable and sever my unity with all ages. I choose to be affirmative and grateful. So, when I watch my grandchildren at play or soccer players speeding down the field, I take pleasure in vicarious participation. I am in them, exuberant for all it means to them and once meant to me.

In spite of Aging's theft, all life is one. I see that more clearly than before. When I bestow a blessing upon youth I am also blessing my life. I only hope that when they are old, they will bless the young.

January 23

Retirement is supposed to free us up to do the things we most need to do, to be the persons we most want to be. Mixed in with that are the obligatory gestures of social membership. Earlier the gas tank was regularly filled, one good night's sleep was sufficient for one whole day of strenuous activity. With Parkinson's, however, with the drain upon me I barely have enough motive power to get through a day, let alone to fulfill the built-in social expectations.

Does Parkinson's Disease give permission to withdraw from normal activities? I struggle to do what once I did eagerly. Now comes the question of what I have a right to dismiss from my social agenda. I have fallen so far behind Vada in what I can bear. I look for a permission slip to be excused from what I earlier wanted to do, but now draw back from. I find myself in a dispute between what is in the fuel tank and how much weight the vehicle can carry.

January 24

In the gap between the affliction and the caretaker resides potential tension. Is it a question of what Vada has a right to expect of me and what I should demand of myself? How did I draw the line between expectation and capacity? The past two days have been very demanding, relative to Parkinson's drag.

Saturday was the funeral of a valued colleague, plus the luncheon following. More and more suffering social aversion, I found the discomfort of social engagement excruciating. When Vada left me in the lurch, I holding her purse, a terror approaching dread overcame me. I felt abandoned. What took me to such a tight place, desire or expectation?

The Saturday before we attended the 50th birthday party of our daughter-in-law, in a crowded room and with an extremely high decibel combo, I was nearly paralyzed upon entrance. My body was present, but my soul had departed. In this cleavage of my self was an almost unbearable torture. My only recourse was to find a quiet corner where I could converse one-on-one, in the effort to save my soul. In leaving I felt a release from hell.

The following day I entered another compression chamber of my own doing, a Peace Meal after the church service. As co-chair of the group I was largely responsible for the organization and the conduct of the occasion. From the beginning I felt a detachment. When I rose to speak, for only a few minutes, I encountered what might be called an out-of-body experience. My identity was somewhere else and I felt a hollowness of existence.

"Why am I here and not somewhere else," I asked myself. "Because I believe in peace," I replied. Then, why was there such a disparity of belief and presence? I realized in that moment that there are some things I can no longer do for peace.

But how do I explain this to others? Yesterday, Sunday, I had a very full schedule with Sunday School, Worship Service, and an afternoon annual meeting of Lancaster Interchurch

Peace Witness, of which I am a Board Member. By the end of the day I was drained, depleted of motivation, stressed and filled with a trembling nervousness. I was glad that the day had come to an end, more than satisfied with a sense of accomplishment!

Now, on a Monday, I am confronted with the prospects of attending the funeral of a church member, years ago the elementary teacher of our children and the wife of a former Treasurer of the College. "What obliges me to attendance," I pondered.

Vada thinks it is the socially considerate response, therefore, expected. Admittedly, she desires my accompaniment as a lifetime spouse. But our capacities are so much different in measure. She assumes what she is able to do, I am also capable of. At what point do I confront the reality of a diminished schedule? Which social engagements, which concerts, which parties, which funerals—which of any events am I to fulfill? And, which do I have a right to decline, in obligation to myself?

As Parkinson is my companion, I know that more and more this will be a pressing question. While not yet benched, I am increasingly on the sidelines. It is no longer a question of wanting to, but the discomfort factor of perhaps not being able to.

January 25

All right, Parkinson, sit down! We have to talk. Earlier I said you had no answers, but I insist on interrogating you nevertheless. Is my life effectually over? Is the rest of life merely a test of will and a measure of suffering's endurance? I accept my share of human suffering, even acknowledging a very fortunate dealing of life circumstances. I hold to the virtue of patience and gratitude. But you are wearing me out!

Is my depression due to the weakening of my body's resilience, or the emotional impact of realizing my future has limited possibilities? I have gone emotionally flat. Parkinson, you have stolen my capacity to care passionately, one of the gifts I valued most.

January 26

Friends, when learning of my Parkinson's diagnosis, say there are no visible signs to indicate the disease. If only they knew what is going on inside! At this stage in Parkinson's, with the aid of medication, the tale is told within. I am hesitant to dwell upon it.

Still, I do not want the experience to go unrecorded, thus, this journal. It helps to have a few others understand, thus a support group. What about my close friends?

February 1

So, the dreary month of January is over. But now I sit in the midst of a crippling winter storm, combining snow and ice into treacherous travel. We are homebound, shut-ins. Something about this external situation strikes me as symbolic of my internal state of affairs. Spring will come again to the world, but will my life from now until death remain January?

February 2

Whether, or not, the groundhog sees its shadow today, a long shadow of gloom has come over me. Yes, we are to live for today, not "fret about the morrow." However, the prospects of the "morrow" are progressively dimming. Unlike with sprained ankles, of which I have had scores, or the multiple cases of flu I have endured, with Parkinson's there is no healing, no getting better. Only prudent management is possible.

I do know the spiritual cure: To grow larger in love of others. If God is Love, there is meaning in Teilhard Chardin's words, *"God is emptying us out, to make room for the Sacred."* My prayer is, do not permit Parkinson to take empathy from me! The worst fate would be to slip into a grave of self-pity.

February 4

Today is my granddaughter Meredith's birthday. I sent her a gift card to buy books. Of course, the gift was to approve of and encourage a love of language. At a deeper level, however, I am blessing the future of my grandchildren. My life is diminishing; may theirs prosper. I do not consider this depression, rather a blessing, traceable to a life instinct. Bless you all, my treasured heirs. May you inherit the Kingdom of Love.

February 6

In terms of Kübler-Ross's stages of accepting death, it seems that I have readily enough by-passed and advanced beyond the first, which is denial. Admittedly, the acceptance has been more cognitive, than existential. As to Parkinson, his presence is amply verified by the body's messages.

In this illness's attendance the question has shifted from the abstract to the inevitable, increasing the emotional voltage. Rather than being angry with Parkinson, I am more annoyed. Maybe it is that in my ninth decade I cannot borrow upon the principle of fairness.

How much right does one person have to ask more of life? Life has been so full, so much. But now, my future has become the past. And I embrace what life has been. *"The future of old age is the past."*

February 9

It is one year since I was diagnosed with Parkinson's. I shall make an assessment: Though only relatively slight, the progression is discernable. The ineluctable course will continue until Parkinson has me in the grip of infirmity. All I can do is to care for myself, as responsibly as possible—take medication, exercise regularly, rest frequently, and maintain a positive attitude.

I am on a low dosage of Sinemet (only a half tablet, four times a day) and some of the symptoms are more pronounced. I seem to be bouncing above and below the desirable level of intake. I only hope that there is not a gradual decrease in effectiveness, requiring increased amount. I am willing to undergo the discomforts for the long-term benefits.

At this stage in Parkinson's progression the symptoms are more internal than visible to others. Last month when I told a long-term acquaintance of the diagnosis, he replied, "You don't show any signs."

However, I undeniably experience symptoms within. Aside from the loss of smell and taste some fifteen years ago, the first real—and very clear—indication came with a trip to Ireland in March two yeas ago, when I felt weak, unable to walk any distance without dragging my feet, especially the right foot.

That fall I had difficulty in carrying my camera equipment, particularly the heavy night lens, out to the soccer field. Being of a somewhat proud (should I say stubborn?) nature, I said that I shall continue with the team so long as I can carry my own gear. If someday confined to a wheelchair, oh how that will have to change!

Not obvious from the outside, Parkinson certainly has taken up residence inside of me. I could regard him as a squatter, on premises that do not belong to him, shouting, "Get off my land!" But that would not lessen the effects or improve my condition.

Ameliorating the discomfort is my main work. The leading disagreeable effects are sharply diminished enthusiasm, an almost constantly present drowsy headache, a sense of futility, and mindfulness of death. Each evening I suffer aching in my feet and ankles, especially the right one, which may be circulation problems related to age more than neurological. Sometimes I feel like a bottle filled with aggravating nervousness. Then, I remember, *Exercise, Exercise, Exercise!*

February 10

The year has been plagued by a sense of futility, a depression of spirit. Depression is a common attending effect of Parkinson's, but I believe a large part of it is psychological—

more attributable to the psyche than to the body (not that they are divisible). It has taken a year to recover from the stunning blow of being diagnosed. Like an incessant gnawing, day and night I am dealing emotionally with readjusting my identity, my life, my future.

It has not been a year wasted, nor am I willing to put the reality of my condition aside, assuming a blithe attitude of feigned lightheartedness. No, I go on with limited facility, yet with a deepened appreciation of life (if that is possible!).

Concomitantly, both ultimacy and gratitude are rising within. With greater earnestness I have a reason to exist (as if I did not before!). Odd, isn't it, greater urgency with lessened capacity. Heightened appreciation in the face of diminishing prospects! How very strange is this thing called "life." What are we to make of it, if not an ongoing course in wisdom?

February 12

It has been thirty-three years to the day of my mother's death. I feel I am carrying on her life in mine. I think not so much of her particulars, as the line of life we both represent. My parents live on in me, just as I will live on in my children and grandchildren. In that, Parkinson, I take some comfort. Looking further down the road of life, I choose tenderness and generosity, a supreme gift to life. Time, indeed, is precious, all for the purpose of giving. That is what true blessing means. We bless by giving of ourselves.

February 14

For Valentine's Day I am going to call a moratorium on talking to Parkinson. I simply have been giving him too much time and attention! This day is for young hearts and sweet sentiments. I choose to join them. Yet, with the water of many years passed, I stand on the other side of the river, smiling upon amorous glances and the coupling of lovers' hands. Having fulfilled my cup of love's potion, I bless them. In the eye of wisdom I have found the sentiment of age.

February 15

Some stages of life cannot be anticipated with reason or "common sense." Such logic would assume, with declining years comes a decrease in valuing of life. Yes, the energy dissipates and, very naturally, motivation is a disappearing impetus, until at last one gently lies down to eternal sleep. But even with limited capacities, I feel the immeasurable privilege of having lived, of being alive. May my daily song be worthy of my worship of life.

February 18

Physically I am on the mend, recovering from my prostate procedure and an unrelenting cold. Slowly I am regaining my strength. However, the verdict remains. I am on a downward course. One can get over a cold, be cured of cancer. But Parkinson's is for the rest of my life. Not "terminal" in immediate terms. Yet, like death itself, always waiting in the wings.

Much I can do to take care of myself—exercise, rest, and medication. But I will not get better. Without cynicism I must accept this. After twenty it is all downhill. The mark of good grace is to absorb this while maximizing purposeful living. The "better" is in wisdom and love. As the body goes down, my soul's character is to go up.

March 3

Well, Parkinson, it has been a while since we talked. Not that I have not thought of you, for you are ubiquitous, always hanging around, ever present in effects. Still, I have decided to "get on with it." You are a dull enough fellow that the conversation soon turns to weariness. Though I can learn from you I prefer not to obsess over you. Too many other important matters lie before me, waiting to be attended to.

And as I attend to those commitments, fortuitously your grip on me seems to diminish somewhat, triggering a return of life desire. Surprisingly, I am happier than one would expect and I enjoy the merriment of good humor. Maybe it is the anticipation of spring, the season of renewal. But is that not a symbol of life's latent energies, the *joie de vivre* springing eternally from the human breast? I am eager to take each day to its maximum. Has that not been my life strategy throughout?

March 4

It is all too apparent, my travels with Parkinson have reinforced important life lessons. "Life is real; life is earnest: and the grave is not its goal." Life is for the living; living is for loving. This reminder makes it clearer that as the years grow shorter, the yearning for life grows greater. Oh, Life, how I embrace you! Not just the future, for I have little of it left. But, rather, the whole of life! That requires a mystical union with totality.

March 7

Parkinson, you have stolen the spring in my step and lessened the passion of my heart. In their place you have left wobbly legs and diminished motivation. Long ago you took from me a sense of taste and smell, followed by my elegant cursive handwriting, now so minuscule that I can barely read it, wobbly like my walk.

Inch by inch, nerve by nerve you have progressed, so that my bright-eyed optimism, my vibrant zest for living has been reduced to a cloudy drowsiness, a perpetual dull headache. Yet I refuse to give in to your demands, not until the day I can no longer say, "Yes" to life. As long as there is an ounce of love in me I shall fight! Not so much in defiance of you, as in honor to having been born.

March 23

OK, Parkinson, Old Boy, again it has been quite a while, the longest since I began this journal of our familiarity. It is not that I have been deliberately avoiding you, for your daily presence is undeniable, so evident in the losses I feel and the symptoms limiting me. Especially with the advent of Spring I have been about other things. One thing I have decided is that **I am not you!** You may be an accomplice, but you are neither the definition of me nor the grand sweep of my life.

So, who are you? Clearly you are neither a friend nor an enemy. More in the order of a "circumstance," a more prominent one of the many life has dished out, you challenge my life urges. And in this test of will, before heaven and earth, I choose the purposefulness of life. I know there will come a time when the weight of physical entropy will become so great that I will resign myself to extinction. That is not life's greatest tragedy. That misfortune would be never having said "Yes" to life.

March 24 [A footnote to yesterday]

Over a half year ago, at a meeting of the evening Parkinson's Support Group, a man well advanced in PD earnestly, yet in a playful spirit, advised me, "Let Parkinson's take care of itself. Get on with life." That was a breakthrough for me, even though I was still in the midst of the necessary grief attending the initial year of diagnosis. Now with Spring, I am all the more resolved to grasp onto what life has yet to offer, rather than dwelling on what is being taken from me.

The physical is diminishing; at the same time opportunity for emotional and spiritual enrichment remains. Love, service, and worship are no less the *raison d'être* of my existence. I shall reach out to each day. Along with this blessing I shall bathe in the sentiment of my entire life. These last chapters of my life will be filled with gratitude for what has been and a relishing of the memory of good moments past.

Each day presents a multitude of moments to reclaim emotional treasures: rain upon my umbrella during a morning walk; birds chirping in the trees of a sunny day; the strains of an English folk melody. Every one releases a flood of heartwarming sentiment. In this is the worship of being alive. Yes, a purpose for living. "Long Live Spring!"

March 25

And now I am back in the conversation in a flurry. What compels writing is the theme: *The Second Year of Diagnosis.* The first year was one of grieving; the second one a new lease on life. I do not believe I was in a strong state of denial, other than to wonder whether there might not be a lessening of the symptoms, given medication. I rather straightforwardly accepted the verdict, being the realist that I am. (Yes, a sentimental romanticist and a dreamy-eyed lover, but in spite of that, a hard-nosed realist.)

The year was spent in absorbing the losses brought by PD and renegotiating my contract with life. Acceptance is a correlative to purpose. And purpose there certainly is, to propel my life forward. Is not life a continuous reevaluation, based upon ability and purpose? Therein lies my new lease on life. Before me is placed a choice: To either drag my feet in complaint or to step ahead as nimbly as possible.

There really is no choice. Until the day my body can no longer carry my soul, I shall choose life. Otherwise, in accord with a lifelong conviction, I would begin dying before I am dead.

March 26

Parkinson, how many ways do I dislike you! (Strange that I should make this my next entry in the ongoing conversation, after having abjured negative complaining. However, I do not regard this exercise so much as complaining as recognition, an inventory of what I have to negotiate. Please see it for the affirmative gesture it intends.) You stole from me at an early meeting my sense of smell and taste. I adjusted quite well to that, regarding those as the least of the five senses. Though I have held food as an aesthetic pleasure, so much of enjoyment is mental and that remains. Having had so many years of enjoyment I can still fancifully imagine the taste of fresh strawberries and the smell of a newly cut Christmas tree.

Then, seemingly picking on my passionate need to write you reduced my penmanship down to tiny, nearly illegible scribble. The dexterity of my fingers has declined to the point that I button sleeves with difficulty, and tremble at the attempt to dial my cell phone. You have all too quickly made a feeble old man out of me!

You have complicated my eating habits with persistent constipation. I now choose food, not for remembered fondness or hedonistic delight, rather in consideration of successful passage.

Into my body you have poured a nervousness beyond what others see or can appreciate. Some days, especially at times of my medication's downswing, I feel like a container of jitters, a bottle of anxiety. You wear me out and put my system in a "shut-down" mode. And when I get up from a needed nap, you leave me feeling as though I have the flu.

Yes, I am even going to hold you responsible for what I have called "social aversion." A reluctance at social engagement has plagued me for years. Crowded places and noisy venues are nearly unbearable. A dread haunts my outgoing nature. Added to this is a wobbliness in gait and an unsteadiness in balance, emanating from a drowsy headache.

Attempts at thinking in pursuit of writing more and more are a venture through a fog of short-term memory fading. I no longer have the confidence to lead a classroom discussion. Yet, the need to contemplate meaning and to articulate understanding persists. I have lost the high point of my mental powers. Still, maybe in consolation, my comprehension and appreciation of wisdom is greater.

Yes, I have lost much, but much remains. There is no other option than to accept that as the condition of my future. With gratitude I take what I still have, for it is all I have a right to ask for. But no thanks to you, Parkinson. I go on, in spite of you, not because. I indict you, yet will not despise you. That would only increase the disquietude. More than anything I desire serenity, filled with love for life.

March 28

A resurgence of purpose occurred at Parkinson's Support Group this evening. An upbeat video left a positive effect upon me. In its twenty minutes a new lease on life emerged. A series of persons testified to years of coping with the disease. Their positive affirmation extended the possibilities for my own life.

For me, a sense of imperative projected into the future. Anticipating another soccer season, I resolved to buy a better camera, a symbolic gesture of forward looking. I said to myself, "You should have bought it last season!" But I thought that was my last one. Night photography has been fraught with difficulty and frustration, the current camera inadequate, stubborn in its auto focusing. This year may well be my last, but I am not going to be bound by that. I am going forward, just like the afflicted on the video.

Anxious about telling Vada of my intentions, I carefully laid out a justification. I had told the Support Group that it is important to have a purpose for each day, in order to look forward. Indeed, looking forward is none other than picking up each day. It is certainly more than a camera, for the camera is only an icon of my regained purpose. Much of my identity has come to be intertwined with my soccer association. The two go together, understanding Parkinson's and finding a purpose to combat it. Along with family and friends, I set myself to "serve them all my days."

March 29

Parkinson, I wish Vada could meet you. Not as a companion, rather to understand what you are like. She is a good and caring person, more so than most. Yet, she has only a telltale idea of what it is to suffer you on an on-going basis. I think she tries, but your presence is an "outside view," based upon what is most real in her affairs of life.

She presumes too much, borrowing upon the earlier me and ordinary expectations. She has accepted the diagnosis, but is slow or reluctant to take into account the affliction. Not intending to be insensitive, the consequences of Parkinson's sometimes exceed her awareness and she asks more of our relationship than is real. She *knows* I have difficulties, *not how hard it is* to do some things.

Understanding this disparity is the very purpose of Caregiver Support Group. Half is instructive; half empathetic. I do acknowledge that she wants to see improvement for my sake, as well as hers.

April 9

Yes, I have not been writing in the journal recently. It is not that I have been inactive, only that I have been concentrating on other areas of thought. Not that I have ignored thinking about my health. On that subject I am in continuous conversation with my body. Today was a down day. Way down. I suspect it qualifies as depression. But it is more so a near total lack of motivation and absence of feeling.

Along with that I have discovered a possible coronary problem. My distal reading has elevated, hovering around 90. Accordingly I made an appointment with the doctor. A little short of panic I pondered how much I may be able to do, including mowing the lawn and traveling with the soccer team.

Health issues are closing in on me. To what extent is the lethargy related to you, Parkinson? I do know that the two, my mortality and you, are inextricably connected. My Parkinson's is another name for senescence, making me all the more aware of my mortality.

April 24

Day of Resurrection. Parkinson's has its own Via Dolorosa and Golgotha. If one is willing to yield up the normal aspirations of life, they are given back with newness. Resurrection is of the spirit, after being wearied by crucifixion of the body. Without the agony of physical affliction, the plateau of normalcy lacks higher appreciation. Each year Parkinson's takes a little more from me. With each resurrection prospects are narrowed. But the wisdom of it all shines more beautifully.

May 1

Walpurgis Nacht → *May Day.* The chilling night of Winter has given way to the glory of Spring. Spring is the time in the life cycle for the spreading of Nature's green carpet, leading to the broad fields of Summer. Every Spring is a time of rebirth, a fountainhead of longing. Nonetheless this year, all the more so. The life spirit still flows, only with greater poignancy. Now I am pained by the thought of how few springs remain. With untrammeled courage I shall go forth once again, to rejoice in life.

May 2

Good news, to go along with Spring! Out of concern for occasional chest throbs last week I was fitted with a Holter monitor to wear for twenty hours. Then, today I got news that my heart is "normal." Oddly, "normal" was a welcomed report, for it carried with it an extraordinary relief. With a long history of heart problems in my male lineage, I felt good fortune in being reassured of my heart's faithful beat.

I had wondered whether Parkinson's was finding just another way to steal from me. There is a frequency of pacemakers among Parkinson's patients. For now, I will be able to set my normal pace, to go forward in an even more appreciative state of mind and spirit.

May 3

For a space of about a month—most of April, my favorite month, my entries have been sporadic, at times nearly sputtering to a stop. It is not that I have not been writing. In fact, typical of Spring's claim upon me I have been inspired to write. During the interlude of April I was able to complete a booklet of religious confession, all written within two weeks' time, to stand once again at the portal of ultimate meaning. It was not as though I had become unaware of Parkinson, for his presence all the more impels the earnestness of my words. Should I thank him, for what I otherwise would not have done?

May 4

In retrospect of the recent past I observe that the more engaged I am in other things, the less attention I give Parkinson. The less I think of him, the less I talk with him. I have, in consequence, accomplished a host of things. Undeniably I am aware of Parkinson's presence. But not dwelling upon it. The relationship is more one of acknowledging someone's presence in the corner of the room, the two of us occasionally directing remarks to one another.

Parkinson is always within me, affecting my every day, but we are not sitting beside each other in a tête-á-tête love seat.

Yes, we are in private conversation, but at a discrete distance. This is so like life and the inevitability of death. The more involved you are with life, the less you think about mortality. But, oh, how quickly the time goes, when fully engaged in living. In opening the moment to death, Parkinson, there is a transcendence of time. A *Tod und Verklärung*, Death and Transfiguration.

May 5

I just finished with my mile walk. Since exercise is stressed in slowing the advance of Parkinson's, I have committed myself to walking a mile as many mornings as possible, rain or shine, umbrella or shorts, cold weather or fair. This walk is preceded by some stretching exercises and arm weight lifting. All of this comes naturally, for life has taught me that exercise is the best toner and energizer for physical wellbeing. Having instilled the practice over many years, I find myself stretching spontaneously, without conscious effort. It is all very natural.

However, while walking used to be a pleasure, now it is a chore. I recall days of hiking miles and miles, nearly effortlessly—out into the country as a boy, along the Rhine River as a man. I would go until I exhausted my body, never more so than after hours and hours of pick-up basketball, incessant running end-to-end on the court. I thrived on it, relished it. Yes, when it was over I was left fatigued and sore, but ever so naturally, the energy willingly spent.

Now, with age taking from me my stamina and Parkinson's weakening my strength, exercise is a triumph of will, not a physical pleasure. Once a "Chariot of Fire," now a broken-down old horse, dizzy and wobbly I go on! Steadfastly must I carry Age and Parkinson with me every step of the way. Is that not some tribute to life, as well as a mark of character?

May 27

Parkinson, why have I not written to you for twelve days? It is not as though I have been trying to get away from you, for I know you will be hanging around until I die. Is it that I have written about all there is to write about my new options in life, attempting to avoid being redundant? Or is it that I do not want to be seen as a chronic complainer, dwelling upon all the down sides to your persistent presence?

I do believe I have "normalized" my life to some extent, having adjusted to what is required for "coping." Besides, I do not care for the renegotiation to dominate my life or to be the sole reason for my existence. Taking my son, John, his wife, and children out to breakfast this morning—a delightfully positive time—reaffirmed what is the real purpose in going on with life. Family and friends have become even more important. The vitality and enthusiasm of my grandchildren transferred a joy into this old heart.

I want much of me to go on living in them. That transfusion will take much time and talk. They like to talk to me and I love to listen. Like all children, they want to grow up. Listening to them, looking them in the eyes while they are talking is more of a grandfather blessing, than lecturing to them. Maybe that is the best way to pass on my life, the greatest gift I can give them.

Parkinson's intensifies the attentiveness, yet must not become a distraction. How wonderful, to have grandchildren who trust me enough to share themselves in talk, with eagerness in their voices and affection in their manner. It makes me want to forget about Parkinson, all the more to listen to them. I told them I felt like the luckiest person in the world.

The last two days I worked hard outdoors, near to the point of exhaustion. Strangely, I feel all the clearer in mind, ready to resume writing, the usual persistent drowsy headache less noticeable. Seemingly, the more purpose, the less the effects. All the more I am convinced at the physical level, along with medication, rest, and diet, exercise is essential to maintenance. Psychologically I need to engage that which is most important to my life.

May 28

Once I did things because I wanted to, driven by the overflowing energy of my body. Now I do what needs to be done, whether or not I want to. My body does not readily respond to the call to walk a mile in the morning or gladly leap to the appointment of a meeting. With lower energy and social aversion I go reluctantly to the theater or symphony. Rather than my body leading the way into action, it is by dint of will power, the invocation of my spirit, that I stumble on my way.

Yet, for all the effort required, I know it would be worse off if I gave in to what Parkinson inclines me not to do. More than ever, it must be spirit over body. My body (legs) put the kite into the air; the uplift of spirit carries my physical shell onward.

June 2

Well, old Fellow, now it is June and soon will come another solstice. Once again nature has spread its broad carpet of green, welcoming all to explore its wonders. But, one year further into aging, I am left with less lust for wandering. I must learn to rely increasingly upon the telescopic lens of memory, while I necessarily distance myself from direct engagement.

In the process I am transitioning to a quieter life style,

hopefully accepting loss more gracefully and appreciating small things more finely. Never exorbitantly selfish, I have begun the work of reconciling myself to mortality. Given the nature of the world I have lived in—endlessly changing and mutating, it seems excessive to expect to live far beyond an average life span. So, as earlier features of life are gradually taken from me, I vow not to curse life.

Rather, I will value the magnificence of what has been and will try to grasp more worshipfully the remaining grandeur. Be that no more than the cool breeze of a morning walk, the awaiting of birth in a Hummingbird nest, or listening attentively, gratefully to the eager talk of a granddaughter, even a less can be a more.

June 3

Is it not enough, Parkinson, that I resist demands upon my ability to do things when my organizational skills have become dulled? Even greater is the loss of processing thought. That, too, requires organization and effort toward a conclusion. My short-term memory is failing and, thus, the chain of thought experiences ellipses. Some days when I attempt to think, it is as though I am stumbling through a thick cloud of undifferentiated objects. Oh, for the days when my mind was clear as a bell.

June 13

More than earlier could have been expected, I have dealt with Parkinson's limitations, subdued the aggravation, and have gone on with the business of living. Life requires purpose, all the more with Parkinson's. In the recovery from the initial blow to my sense of purpose, I have rediscovered my role in life, even more advanced: The Stage of Grandfather Blessing. Having last week visited five of my grandchildren, in Allentown and Annapolis, I see more clearly the role life has now assigned me: To affirm the worth of those that come two generations after me. I am also all too aware that this is a desire to extend my own life into the future. The span from my birth to the death of my last surviving grandchild will likely be 150 years!

Parents have the sometimes not too pleasant responsibility of setting the boundaries for the young, even during the tumultuous time of adolescence breaking loose amid confusion and rashness. I, on the other side of the generation divide, have the enviable task of saying nice things about my grandchildren. Though their pace is too swift and the noise much too disconcerting, I genuinely like them and see goodness in their being. It makes this all the more satisfying having developed a trusting relationship with them.

They truly like me and prosper in the acceptance/ affirmation I bless them with. They glow when I tell them they are "super great" in my eyes. Parents take care of the mischief; I, the elder of the clan, bless. So, Parkinson, you may have your hand on me, but I still have a purpose with which to go on. Necessarily, though, I will take good care of me—exercise and medication—I will concentrate more on my purpose, than on you!

July 4

Much has happened in the three weeks since the last entry. Most significant was the 1,250 mile trip to Kansas, to join with Vada's family in a reunion. While it is not likely the last major overnight journey for me, still it made me all the more aware of how much I have lost from the combination of Parkinson's and aging.

I have become increasingly anxious about speed and destination. What was once routine problem solving is now a worrisome task. I resist new challenges and sustained mental activity. Reading has become wearisome, my eyes blurry and my attention fuzzy. But most troublesome has become my low level of motivation. Some days approaching lassitude, my life impulse lapses into inertia. A sense of life purpose comes and goes, some days lost in depression. Then I feel the onus of life wasted, a betrayal of life's greatest gift, gratitude.

For causes I do not comprehend, on the very next day

comes a resurgence of desire and I justify my existence with a small burst of creativity. However, it is all too evident overall that my life is in sharp decline. All I ask is that I preserve dignity and a positive disposition.

July 18

Either summer heat is taking a toll on me or Parkinson's is a bit more advanced. I am tired most of the time and motivationally listless. A state of languor has set in. Anxiety persists, creating mild dread when a date requiring public responsibility approaches. Fret arises. Will I be able to sustain another soccer season, physically and emotionally? Unfortunately, stress exaggerates some of the symptoms.

Yesterday, watching the Women's World Cup—U.S versus Japan—a nervousness came over me, a quivering from inside. What will it be like during suspenseful soccer games this fall? My wiser counsel tells me to let what will be, be, but my body takes on the condition of nervousness.

Also, I notice that I am losing arm strength. After holding up my upper body while reading I felt my arms tremble. That certainly is related to Parkinson's. Should I ask for an increase in medication dosage the next time I see my neurologist? I am quite convinced that the Sinemet is what produces the side effect of drowsy headache. It is a discretionary call, symptom versus side effect. I also am told that the medication increases dizziness and loss of balance. I no longer can rely upon nature taking care of me.

July 30

As alternating current, the life force comes and goes. I am in another period of low motivation and increased depression. I force myself to get up and walk, knowing that exercise will improve my disposition and that I will feel worse if I don't. Little things have a disproportionate effect upon me. Major difficulties nearly paralyze me.

A scratch on the door of Vada's new car, incurred through a misjudgment in driving into the garage, glares at me as an accuser. We were returning from Annapolis and I was weary. Vada assigns some of the fault to my problematic left eye. But the damaged door jeers at me with each glance, taunting my ability to drive. I cannot see the beauty of a luxurious car, only the blemish.

This is so characteristic of Parkinson's anxiety. The image slips into my dreams and haunts my days. Along with this are all the demands imposed upon me, stressing my will power. I have a limited capacity to manage and organize. At a certain point I feel overwhelmed and then shut down.

Is it fair of me to tell family and friends that I cannot bear the load once normally expected, by me as well as them? I know I have lost the ability to care physically for my grandchildren. The constant attention required is too much. Slowly I am being reduced down to what is essential in the process of conducting everyday affairs and, that with reduced motivation, I am set off from the others in my life.

August 6

I have been avoiding writing, not because of other things, but because I am psychologically down. So much—U.S. financial credit, politics in general, doubt about the return of an outstanding soccer player, worry over family matters, on and on—seems to be going wrong.

Parkinson's is just one more big concern! It brings depression and that only makes me less motivated, which depresses me all the more. Not only do I not want to write, I even avoid typing my script into the computer. I am really down because I realize all too well that the way to go on is to have important things to do, projects and people I care about. Otherwise I would be inert.

August 9

Here on my birthday I look back at many years of life. To where has time brought me? It has been altogether a good life, filled with love and beauty. Yet, a milestone has been reached. To a large degree the joy has drained out; day-to-day existence has become a struggle. No longer do I have the capacity to enjoy what once were the ordinary pleasures.

A drowsy headache persists, my gait is wobbly, and my left eye has developed ghostly double images, making reading tiresome. I exist much of the time in a thick cloud of mental haze. It is difficult to focus attention on what is going on around me. The genius of writing visits me less and less. I realize that my best years of thought and writing are over.

I still gratefully hold life in my hands, not with the easy enthusiasm of youth but with diminishing vitality. It has been a very gradual descent into infirmity, for which I am thankful. Here I am, finding that my relationship to life, my general outlook, has been significantly altered. It is a strange, rather surrealistic existence I confront. Thank you life, for all that you have been. May that sustain my spirit to the end.

August 12

Parkinson, are you merely a bad dream, from which I shall someday awaken, a hallucination which will eventually go away? I exist in an alien land, strange to myself and unfamiliar with the terrain. It is as though another person has taken over me, one that I scarcely know. This person does not have the predisposition I once had. Always introspective, now I am much more inward, groping to find the reason for my existence. Must I learn all over again who I am, how to walk the daily path?

August 29

A second soccer season since diagnosis, most clearly my last. I feel as though I am revisiting all the twenty seasons simultaneously. The anticipation has been both anxious and a quickening of my step. My spirit still responds to the call, but doubts arise as to how well I can keep up the pace. I struggle with drowsiness and dragging motivation, yet it seems as if I am outpacing Parkinson.

As can be seen in the lull in writing, I have not been conversing much with him. Still, he is right behind me and I know he will eventually catch up with me. In the meantime I will devote myself to the aspirations of youthful soccer players. Little does youth understand the effects upon me by Parkinson, our worlds quite distant from one another. Nevertheless, I exist in both, remembering the days of vitality while afflicted by aging.

August 31

The end of August has come and my kid brother turns seventy-five! What does this mean, if not that the end of the road is coming closer? The cooler weather, thanks to the aftermath of a hurricane, marks a turning of the corner into autumn, the season of life's restful return to the earth! Toward the end, life is a blur of all days lived. A mellowness captivates me. Sentimental about the past, embracing the whole of life, I walk in the golden glow of remembrance.

May I look forward to another spring, the season of renewal, or am I to glory in the reverie of autumn? Once I lived mainly in the present; now my life has filled out to all-encompassing goodness. Even though Parkinson will accompany me to the end of the road, I have made some progress in accepting that as my assigned fate. The consolation is that Parkinson cannot take away from me the sentimental hours of remembrance. In that I have triumphed over him.

October 13

Such a long time and most of a soccer season has passed. Busyness brushed you aside, Parkinson. But now you have a competitor! It is called a stroke, about which I am learning through direct experience. Parkinson, you took my right side into weakness, now my right side is under the siege of numbness. Both of you leave me a little more unstable on my feet.

Again I am challenged to affirm the will to live. Rather than concentrating on what I have lost in health, I look at each day as a new opportunity for which to be grateful. More than ever consciousness amazes me. I shall never more take it for granted.

October 26

I do want to get back to more regular writing. Time is precious and recording my late life experience is a priority. I still reminisce over the goodness of life, the moments filling me with a sense that I have lived well. But a growing urgency has come to the center of my daily living. My health has undergone significant enough decline, that I take even more seriously preparations to say good-bye to life. Monday I took over to the College for duplicating the pamphlet that I would like to be used at my memorial service.

Many of the ordinary daily concerns have receded, to be trumped by the ultimate. I no longer make plans for trips or major projects. This is a strange world to negotiate. I have always lived close to ultimacy, what is called "thin places," but this intensified consciousness is overwhelming. I feel that I am entirely in the extraordinary dimension.

October 28

I plod along, more and more the old man. The stroke was almost an "overnight" transformation. Will a cane soon come to join me and Parkinson? My heart, now with some weakness, would go on, but my wobbly balance slows my pace. I relish the days of youth, when my feet were nimble and fast. Now I can only admire vicariously the vitality of youth from the sidelines.

I have personified Parkinson, to facilitate a conversation. It seems a host of personalities have been added to his presence. Altogether, are they not the figure of the Grim Reaper? Better yet, Father Time? Have I not become wise in years? It is not against powers and principalities we contend. Rather, it is Life and Death. Glory in Life, that Death may be merely an event. Either fear in dying, or joy in having lived. The longer I live the greater the richness of my fantasy. Both wise and bent by time, I go on.

October 30

In combination, Parkinson's and the recent stroke have left me in a surrealistic zone between life and death. The outlook on everything has been altered. Life seems receding and death approaching. I think of everything in terms of death. Cautious of over exerting myself, I am hesitant to jump into physical activity, including exercise. Possibly over-attentive to bodily signals, I am anxious about taxing my heart and precipitating another stroke.

Though I have always been very bodily aware, I am now fixed upon my physical decline. Simple tasks, such as getting up to clean off the sidewalk from snow, require extraordinary consideration. I am grateful that the stroke has not left me incapacitated. Yet, every exertion is with greater effort. Even the weather seems surrealistic.

With the snowstorm of yesterday, nearly unprecedented in its early arrival and measure, my world of consciousness is reinforced by physical reality. Tree limbs have fallen in the backyard, but I can do little to clear the damage. Rather than thinking of responsibilities, I dwell upon physical limitation. The storm postponed the last soccer game of the season with Messiah College, ranked number one in the nation, throwing me emotionally into a dither.

My energy, thus my will, has declined. I want to go on. The role I have served for so long is very important to me. But the recalculations required to fulfill the role put me into a state of consternation. More and more difficult is it to readapt to physical necessities. Am I progressively slipping into an inert consciousness, aware but not responding? Is that not a dying out?

November 11

It has been around a century since the original marking of this date. For my own part, I won't make it to the century mark, but I can use the occasion to mark a significant development in life. Growing up we referred to the date as *Armistice Day,* a designation I still prefer. Accepting the more recent name of *Veterans Day,* I shall include myself.

No, not that I "served" in the armed forces. But that I have agonized the pain and human tragedy of war. By empathy and vicarious experiencing I have suffered with the afflicted, even so much as to identify with the injured and dead. Recently I willingly received a black wristband with the inscription, *"Believe in Heroes."* I seek identity with the "fallen." Rather than glorifying warfare, I "feel companion with the dead." There is glory enough in the joy of armistice.

At a mortal level, in a profound sense, I am contending with death. With Parkinson on my right and the touch of Stroke on my left, I am being escorted along the narrowing path toward death. The inevitability of death has deepened the seriousness of life throughout. Now I am ushered into a surrealistic realm in which thoughts of death are predominant, leaving all else secondary.

With declining motivation and energy I am more preoccupied with how little time I have, how I must prepare myself for death, than engaged in the ordinary enjoyment of the present. The balance has shifted. Once the reality of death was remote; now it has taken center stage. All the furniture has been rearranged. Indeed, it is a strange new world!

November 16

And now there are three: Age, Parkinson's, and Stroke. They bear different names, but how do I keep them apart? On many of my afflictions they are in agreement. They all are walking me in the direction of senility. Oddly, as my gait slows, their advance seems to speed up. Of one thing I am certain—the young Gene is vanishing, The Gang of Three shall not steal either my identity or dignity.

November 26

Thanksgiving is over and I have even more to be thankful for. I have lost much, but my gratitude has increased. More so, what I have is even more treasured and of greater value. My family, hectic as the gatherings may be, is an extension of my life.

I shared with my granddaughter Meredith that I live on in the positive influence I can make upon my grandchildren. Though she is young, being precocious and of spiritual kinship, I believe the commendation of my legacy is secure with her. The grandchildren are gone, but the connection lingers on. Even music is of purer quality, as I contemplate the end of life. I defy Parkinson to take that from me.

November 28

I have resumed my morning walks, though dropping back to a mile, from a mile and a half. Like the day itself, from dusk to light, I awaken again. More than a rejuvenation, I speak of a resurrection of spirit as the body comes to life anew. Because of aging and Parkinson's I start out as a bear, still wanting to hibernate. Stiff and a little sore I call upon a higher power to summon my declining life impulse. Little by little, a reluctant step becomes a more open stride, energy begins to trickle back into me. By the end of the walk my wings of desire open and the day lies before me as a welcome. I experience the promise of exercise's regimen.

Exercise, Exercise, Exercise! That has been the resounding acclaim of the medical professionals. Now, I am even more a believer. I may not be able to defeat Parkinson, but I will strive to keep ahead of him on my walk. Parenthetically, Mr. TIA Stroke, my walk seems less wobbly and my sense of balance better.

December 1

And now comes another December, almost a year since I began this journal. In some respects life has once again normalized itself. No, not returned to what it was before, rather adjusted to new development, with the desire to go on under the circumstances.

For most of the year thoughts of Parkinson's dominated the internal conversation. Now, gradually that has shifted to what I still wish to do with my life. One might speak of the process as a rebirth of the life impulse. I know that my time is limited and that only a few years are left. Thus, I am more selective of what is important. The selectivity is more one of culmination, than occupation.

The work of life is nearly over; what remains is a flourish of final touches. In a mixture of nostalgia and urgency, I go on to a benediction of life. It has been good; I revere the thought of it, wanting to combine the best of my remembrance with a nicely wrapped gift for loved ones surviving.

December 13

Parkinson's both decreases the will power and increases the need to act out the meaning of life, a vice grip in which regret is rebuffed and the anvil upon which importance is to be forged. I find a sense of importance inseparable from spiritual survival. If what I am doing does not bear some ultimate significance, the desire to go on living diminishes. Thus, ongoing life becomes an enterprise of creating meaning where little previously existed.

With the craft of alchemy acquired, the crude metal of ordinariness is transmuted into the precious coins of extraordinary living. The empty space of thoughtless existence is interrupted by a powerful impulse to reply to the cosmos with gifts carved out of substance from the soul. That is the essence of importance! What would I do without it? Some days it almost drives me crazy; other days I rest in the assurance that life has been good. Is Parkinson complicit in this madness, or merely a curious by-stander?

December 15

Now, once again, I enter into the intensity which is Christmas. I have since childhood thrived on the thrill a heightened sense of gladness brings. But, over the last decade the tingle has waned, and my weary emotions reluctant to get involved, almost as though fantasy's enchantment can be worn out. The child in me gave way to pretence for the sake of my grandchildren.

This year is different, for enthusiasm has returned. Perfunctory card writing, in gesture to the season, has become opportunity for sincere giving of myself. I am more upbeat, less dour. More willing to make a go of it, rather than merely waiting until quiet returns.

After a year of concern about my health, oddly yet rightly, I find new meaning in old gestures. Parkinson and I have decided to fill the stockings with delicacies. We have limited time here and so many presents to give, before we rest. The greatest loss is realizing that not many Christmases are left.

Thus, with every package goes a blessing. All is wrapped in the bright colors of mirth, tied with a bow of loving tenderness. Christmas is still the high holiday of affection and beauty, a marriage of charity and life's goodness. No ailment, temporary or terminal, should be allowed to take that from me.

December 21

Parkinson has a crony by the name of Depression, or that is what in most cases the affliction is accompanied by. For a lifetime I have been prone to melancholy, but now I am experiencing something quite different. For some months, and more pronounced the last few days, I have been preoccupied by thoughts of death's inevitability. Without any attempt at calculating the days and years left, I am possessed by the end's immanency.

I am somewhat anxious about the health of my heart, even more so than over what Parkinson is doing to me. A catheterization is scheduled for early next year; I am advised not to walk at length, not more than a slow pace. Increasingly I am hesitant to exert myself, even with knowing that inactivity is a path to decline. The quality of life certainly has taken a downward course. Not feeling well—I liken most of my day hours to a dismal state of wobbly drowsiness— and low on motivation, night falls on a day of disappointed accomplishment.

I want to be courageous in accepting the terms of life's conditions. Yet, I worry that I will be swallowed up by a decline in spirit. Always a sentimentalist in the extreme, I am already detecting a de-sentimentalizing of things held dear. If sentiment is, as I have said in my good years, the attachment to the best of life experience, is what I am undergoing a "losening?" An "ungluing?" Without sentiment projected into the future, what we live for and the motive force for "going on" disappears. When death approaches, sadly the sentimental reason for living diminishes. I have never experienced this before. And I do not want to become distraught over it!

Christmas Eve

On this, the Eve of Christmas, how the memories of *Silent Night* and hushed, candlelit services pour in. Probably it is this rite that has meant the most to me over the years, a "thin place" where eternity pokes its solemnity into time. In the distant reach of memory are the first encounters with this timelessness, in company of my family in the First English Lutheran Church, Goshen, Indiana. Later, when we traveled "home" from Pennsylvania, the family grew to include our children. After the renewed encounter with sacred time it was difficult to fall asleep. Not because of the anticipated presents of morning. Rather in consequence of having brushed so close to heaven.

However, I face this year's awe-inducing ceremony with such an altered view of life. For reasons that confuse me, the level of sentiment connected with the holiday season has diminished. Once I poured my entire self into the mystique of the tradition. Now, the emotions have gone flat. Earlier I found it painful to say good-bye to the decorations, carols included. This year I will take down the tree, symbol of all that is lovely and treasured, with little feeling. My overtures to the season are mainly for the sake of the child, still lingering in me and presumed to be alive in my grandchildren.

December 31

The year has come to an end. How do I finish this journal? Significant developments have occurred. How do I measure the progression of Parkinson's? In some respects the year has seemed to pass by quite quickly. Thus, I cannot easily account for all that has happened. Maybe it is because there has been a reduction of my life down to a few concerns for taking care of myself: regularity of medication, frequency of rest, and preoccupation with my health.

The advance of the disease seems only moderate. But I am more and more beset by muscular stiffness and weakness. Some of this I would like to associate with the effect of cholesterol-reducing statins. At times weariness with life takes over; yet, then a restored will to go on returns. Overall, I would certainly acknowledge that there has been a decline in quality of life.

So, how do I welcome a new year? With renewed resolve? Or, further efforts to put final touches on my life story? I do affirm that no matter what lies ahead I vow to keep a positive spirit, to bless others and relish their presence. As I heard recently, "We ought to love those in our life, while we have them."

Should I say, "I want my end to be as high class as the life I have striven to live"? **I have loved it all!**

Pause for a Postscript:

If there were a title to this postscript it likely would be "The Radical Reordering of Life." This episode on my life journey has not been only a meeting with a shadowy figure named Parkinson. Having the disease also means crossing a boundary into a late stage of life. A major shift in the conditions of my existence has occurred.

No longer can some assumptions be made or certain gifts of life be presumed. A clear diminishing of quality has occurred, never to return. Unlike most illnesses, I will not get better. *In for the long haul* is none other than *until death do us part.*

One of the most grievous losses is that of a sense of importance. In youth almost anything fascinated me. Now, little has the power to grasp my interest. It is as though I entered a different realm of being, separating the after from the before.

Am I the same person, or has a somewhat altered me taken Eugene's place? Who am I and why has so much changed? The world is not perceived in quite the same way and why is there a modification in feelings about life? Not a little bewilderment attends my thoughts. I presume this is the case with all major changes in health circumstances when life is pressed to its limit. Nevertheless, this has become my unique story and I take it as my own.

Most regrettable is the decline in zest, that faithful chariot of passion and enthusiasm. Enthusiasm means to be filled with a divine spirit and has been my Song to Life. But diminished is the ardor and quieter the music. How does one love and worship, when the divine energy runs out? Oh, Parkinson, are you a teacher of wisdom, or an irreverent thief?

Closing a Year's Conversation

What is begun is not always what is finished. Such an acknowledgement certainly applies to this journal of reflections. The start of a conversation does not guarantee its ending. Conversation must be as flexible as life itself. Honest reflection is vagrant as well as expansive. True as the adage, "One thing leads to another," day-to-day conversation with life knows no bounds. Unlike most of my booklets, which are held together by a theme logically developed, human thought is endlessly engaged in novelty and discovery. Vital thought is ceaselessly mutating, evolving into what it was not. In tribute to this primal process of thought, no attempt has been made to reorder the discoveries into a watertight tome. I shall permit them to stand as they emerged.

Now having recorded a year of inner thoughts, all the clearer is the association of Parkinson and Death. I realize that my affliction has become a surrogate for my mortality. Thus, though I had intended to limit the conversation to the struggle with the disease, all of life began to pour in, to the profoundest level thinkable. That does not mean "anything goes," however, I really did want to focus on how Parkinson's affected my life. But how does one separate between health and outlook? The eye altering, alters all. And compromise in well-being affects secondary considerations. Even what was central in active years yields to the core of one's existence, the meaning of life and death. How could I keep the very meaning of my existence out of the conversation? As with all earnest reflection, the reason for my existence has become better understood. Is that not the higher purpose in conversing with Death? At least that is what for years I taught my students.

Quite so, in looking back over what I have written I detect a larger outcome than a conversation with Parkinson. Coincidentally, flowing out of the words of narration have come the core values of my life, principally: Acceptance and Affirmation; Gratitude and Giving; Awe and Appreciation. Thus, this journal has been simultaneously a portrait of who I am. The title of writing could be altered to emphasize more the larger picture, but I am content to leave the focus upon my late bout with Parkinson's Disease. I only trust that the reader perceives the dual level of meaning. The effects of the disease could be recorded until the day I die. However, at this point I will draw the particular conversation to a close. A year seems sufficient duration to make the point. I have learned much. The record can be passed on to those who love and survive me. I trust to a few more years. Being an incorrigible writer—because I am an incessant thinker—the reflective conversation with life will go on, to fall into other containers bearing cleverly mind-arresting titles. As long as the life urge remains in me, I shall write.

It is my wish that my bones be returned to the elements that have for so long sustained me. In releasing my individuality will come union with all that is. What good has flowed through me I transfer to those I have been privileged to share life.

I thank my dear lifetime companion, Vada, for her steadfast care and my children, David, John, and Kristina, for their abiding respect. They are the living vessels into whom I have poured my love. Thus, they are forever inseparable from me. Not historically coincident, they are who I am. They have given me far more than Parkinson can ever take from me.

The Five-Year Anniversary of Meeting Mr. Parkinson

Five years now have passed since the last entry in this journal, *but Mr. Parkinson is still with me. In the subsequent years after the diagnosis, I could have continued the inner conversation through periodic writing, marking the progressive losses. Yet, after a year of soul wrestling following the year I wrote my journal, I felt an emotional breakthrough that has had a profound effect on my thinking. Though the infirmity persists, the intensity of needed resolution has given way to the blessing of acceptance which has brought lightness.*

It seems strangely significant to me that, although my symptoms are more debilitating than six years ago, I am more at peace with the conditions of my life than in the earlier stages. Having lost what once were major involvements, I have revised old ones and discovered emerging new ones. The specifics have altered, but the fulfillment goes on. All of life proceeds through a series of phases and this is true as well with Parkinson's.

Odd as it may sound, the greater torment accepting the adverse in our lives may come toward the beginning, rather than toward the end, the assent being dependent on how the reality of aging and death is confronted and dealt with. Call it courage or life affirmation, the fact remains that how loss is spiritually dealt with determines the quality of remaining life. I confess that life is still a tenuous affair, but I believe in the positive and I seek to honor its truth.

We live in the intersection between the dream of our ideals and the harsh reality of intransigent physical limitations. We would that we lived forever, but the facts invade the breech in longing. The resulting turmoil is like unto a storm, replete with emotional reverberations and hoped for flashes of illumination.

Be it noted, however, the objective is not merely to survive the unsettling of life's tranquility. Something qualitatively greater is possible, and that is a spiritual enrichment. In life, as with weather, the calm coming after the storm is fuller and richer than the calm before. Prior to the turbulence we are innocent; after the existential engagement with life's marriage of spirit and body, comes wisdom. Thus, we are driven out of the idealized garden of unlimited desire. But the reward is authenticity.

Never can the tragic be brought into unqualified acceptance because the morally absurd is woven into the very fabric of our lives and the most soul-rending battles are fought within the quandary of life's ambiguities. Trying to justify misfortune through some cosmic principle only adds to the perversity.

Yet, in the face of irreducible irrationality—whether it be Parkinson's or any other major change in one's life—a spiritual transformation can occur. All is dependent upon a "letting go." Once we accept that we cannot command the universe, we can then grant ourselves the peace of acceptance.

EPC

www.ingramcontent.com/pod-product-compliance
Lightning Source LLC
Chambersburg PA
CBHW050606280326
41933CB00011B/1996